Handbook for Intractable Pain

Recognition and Treatment

Forest Tennant
(DrPH, MPH, MD)

Published by the Tennant Foundation
West Covina, California

ISBN: 9781955934329
Library of Congress Control Number: 2023921074

Special discounts are available on quantity purchases by corporations, associations, educators, and others. For details, contact one of the parties listed below.
U.S. trade bookstores and wholesalers: Please contact. Nancy Kriskovich
Tel: (406)249-2002; or
email snkriskovich@gmail.com

All proceeds from the sale of this book will go to the Medical Study and Education Projects sponsored by the

Tennant Foundation
336-338 S. Glendora Ave.
West Covina, CA 91790-3043
Ph: 626-716-2689
Fax: 626-919-7497
Email: tennantfoundation92@gmail.com

ACKNOWLEDGEMENTS

This book could not have been researched and written without the technical assistance of Becky and Tom Marino, Ingrid Hollis and Nancy Kriskovich

DEDICATION

This handbook is dedicated to Kristen Ogden and Red Lawhern for their tireless advocacy on behalf of Intractable pain patients.

Table of Contents

Prologue

The realization that a subgroup of chronic pain patients has Intractable pain and what amounts to a disease is finally spreading. Over half a dozen states now have IP laws and Wikipedia not only defines IP but refers to IP as a disease. At this time persons with IP and their medical practitioners can and must recognize that IP exists and has some specific treatment measures of which many are provided in this handbook.

A major impediment to treatment of IP is simply that it is not being recognized by either patient or practitioner. Basically, the concept that pain, per se, can cause serious medical complications is not yet appreciated. This fact is evidenced in product advertising and lay person media articles about chronic pain. A close analysis implies that everyone has simple chronic pain and needs a "one size fits all" treatment.

The fact is that the IP subgroup of persons isn't usually known to exist or recognized by even the most sophisticated and prestigious medical institutions. For example, I hear almost daily about a person with IP who has severe hypertension, tachycardia, or even angina without any recognition that IP is the culprit. Other examples are persons with IP who have hormonal deficiencies. Medical practitioners are treating their patients for such hormonal complications as osteoporosis, impotence, and depression with no recognition that IP is the cause. Regrettably, some persons have had their pituitary or adrenal removed for a “tumor” when in reality the gland was over functioning and enlarged due to IP.

IP is not a common disease compared to such diseases as diabetes and asthma. Consequently, the health care system often gives persons with IP “short shrift.” This compels the IP person, with the help of their family, to provide much of their own care. The first chapters in this handbook are dedicated to general education about IP. The second section of this handbook is a stepwise program of self-help.

IP doesn’t have to thrust a person into misery and a short life if a three-component protocol is followed: (1) suppression of inflammation and autoimmunity, (2) restoration of damaged tissues, (3) pain control. To carry out this protocol, one has to become knowledgeable about IP and build, over time, an effective therapeutic program.

Introduction

Persons with IP are a subgroup of persons with chronic pain. The hallmark of IP is constant pain. Normal chronic pain comes and goes with remissions and exacerbations. IP is often considered a syndrome or disease because it has multiple causes and complications. Once in place IP causes dysfunctions of many bodily systems. The cardiovascular, endocrine, gastrointestinal, respiratory, and immunologic systems may all malfunction unless IP is controlled. This is done with a three-component protocol: (1) suppression of inflammation and autoimmunity, (2) restoration of damaged tissues, (3) pain control. Failure to adequately control IP not only permits agony, misery, and a ruined life, it shortens a life. To gain control of IP a program of both medical and self-care is essential. This handbook provides general information in its first part, and the second section is a stepwise group of self-help measures. My experience in treating and caring for persons with IP is clear. If the steps described in this handbook are followed, a comfortable, long quality of life is the usual outcome.

What is Intractable Pain (IP)?

Intractable pain (IP) is medically defined as a constant, severe, incurable condition that causes pathologic alterations in the cardiovascular, gastrointestinal, endocrine, immunologic, cerebral, and metabolic systems. Although this condition was recognized by physicians in past centuries, the name intractable was only applied in the twentieth century. Physicians have attempted a variety of treatments over the centuries which included bizarre measures such as electric eels, bloodletting, and brain removal. Only in very recent years has there been an understanding of the development, causes, and treatment of IP. This handbook has been written to help persons with IP, their family and medical practitioners recognize and effectively treat IP.

At its most elemental and biologic level IP is a combination of damaged nerves and inflammation. It only occurs as the end result of one or more pathologic conditions that lead to nerve damage and inflammation. Nerve damage which causes pain is often referred to as neuropathic pain. An appropriate adjective could be inflammatory, neuropathic pain.

Recent discoveries now implicate autoimmunity-in the development of IP. Autoimmunity is when some element in the body such as a toxin or antibody attacks one's own tissue to produce inflammation, nerve damage and pain. A number of viruses, especially Epstein Barr, are now known to produce autoimmunity and inflammation may be a major, causative factor in the development of some cases of IP.

Do You Have Intractable or Chronic Pain?

It is essential that every person with chronic pain recognize if they have IP, because this means that some neurotransmitter-receptor systems in the central nervous system are no longer functioning in a manner that shuts off the pain. Special treatment is required for IP.

The Table presented below shows differences between chronic pain (CP) and IP. A diagnosis of IP should never be applied to a person unless constant pain is present as well as some of its known complications.

	IP	CP
Pain is Constant (24/7)	Yes	No
Treatment is Daily (Around the Clock)	Yes	No
Elevated Blood Pressure and Pulse Rate	Yes	Seldom
Elevated Temperature and Breathing Rate	Yes	No
Anorexia/Malnutrition	Yes	No
Insomnia	Yes	No
Depression, Hopelessness	Yes	No

Endocrine Abnormalities (Hormones & Glucose)	Yes	No
Elevated Inflammatory Markers	Often	Seldom
Restriction of Certain Life Activities (e.g., mobility)	Yes	Sometimes
Decreased Capability for Requirements of Daily Living	Yes	No

After reviewing the above table, it should be clear whether one has IP or CP. Once a person feels they have IP, they need to inform their family and medical practitioners of such. Begin keeping a record of your pulse, breathing rate, and blood pressure. Educate yourself as much as possible. Share written materials you can find on IP. Recall and record in your personal medical records when your condition began and what you believe initiated your condition.

How IP Develops

Thanks to research and studies of recent years, there is now an understanding of the pathologic sequences that lead to IP. Basically, IP is the end product of multiple events and conditions that affect a person. About half of the persons who develop IP have a genetic or inherited disorder. The most common high risk genetic conditions are Ehlers-Danlos Syndrome (EDS), ankylosing spondylitis (AS), and scoliosis. EDS is a connective tissue disorder in which the body, due to a gene defect, fails to produce the quantity or quality of collagen that is necessary to keep bodily tissue strong and resistant to infections and injuries. Ankylosing spondylitis (AS) is a disease which weakens and causes degeneration of discs and fusion of the spine. Other genetic or inheritable, but less common disorders that may cause IP include Marfan Syndrome, porphyria, and autoimmune diseases such as rheumatoid arthritis and ulcerative colitis.

IP always has a starting or painful initiating event which is either: (1) traumatic, or (2) inflammatory. Typically, the initiating event takes place several months or years before IP develops.

The most common traumatic events are falls, altercations, or surgery. Trauma may be to the head, spinal cord, or nerves in the arm or leg. The most common initiating inflammatory disorders are fibromyalgia, severe respiratory infection, or arthritis.

The initiating event doesn't usually cease but "smolders on" with pain that comes and goes. A diagnosis of chronic pain is likely assigned, and a wide variety of medications and other measures are attempted. Interestingly, an initiating inflammatory event such as arthritis or fibromyalgia may seemingly spread. The person may develop additional inflammatory disorders such as thyroiditis, carpal tunnel syndrome, migraine, and irritable bowel.

Trauma may be severe or minor and the sequelae quite variable. Neuropathies or intervertebral disc degeneration and herniations are common traumatic complications that lead to IP. Pain after the initiating event is usually not constant, but, at some point, it becomes constant.

Pain constancy is associated with inflammation that develops in the brain and/or spinal cord (CNS). Cells called glia or microglia promote CNS inflammation which literally damages the neurotransmitter-receptor systems that control pain. Exactly how injuries and inflammatory disorders activate glial cells to produce CNS inflammation is unclear. The two most probable mechanisms are (1) excess electromagnetic energy generated by the injury or inflammation, and (2) autoimmunity or viral invasion of CNS tissue. The Epstein Barr virus is the most likely virus.

The initiating event in the development of IP is either a traumatic injury or inflammatory disorder. The time frame between the initiating event and IP is quite variable. It can range from days to years.

Major Causes of IP

As noted in prior chapters, IP is often called a syndrome or disease. Some observers like to say it is persistent, high impact, or centralized pain. Regardless of past or current adjectives, IP is preferred name and the end product of multiple pathologic developments that precede it. For this reason, a person with IP may be given multiple labels. There are today, however, only a few conditions that cause the great majority of the cases. Here are today's common causes of IP:

Common Causes of IP (2023-24)	
Adhesive Arachnoiditis-Lumbar-Sacral Spine	Arthritis-Severe
Complex Regional Pain Syndrome (CRPS)	Multiple Herniated Discs
Ehlers-Danlos Syndrome (EDS)	Post-Stroke
Arachnoiditis-Cervical Spine	Traumatic Brain/Spinal Cord Injury

It is interesting that some common IP conditions of yesteryear are no longer common since treatments have been developed for the causative disease. Examples are interstitial cystitis, sickle cell anemia, and ulcerative colitis. There are several rare conditions that may cause IP including porphyria, Marfan Syndrome, and hydrocephalus.

Pain You Can Recognize

IP has pain characteristics that are typical, easy to recognize, and quite different from usual, common chronic pain.

First, the hallmark of IP is constant pain. It never goes away except when one is sleeping. What's more, a person with IP will usually have to take a sedative to achieve sleep. Persons who have chronic pain experience periodic or intermittent episodes of pain. For example, a joint or muscle may ache for a few hours or days, and then the pain goes away for a while. Not so with IP. The pain never leaves.

Besides constant pain the person with IP will experience what is called flare or breakthrough pain. This is pain on top of a baseline pain.

Today many physicians like to refer to constant pain as centralized, central, or central sensitization. The new labels have emerged since it is now known that the CNS has been anatomically and biochemically altered to produce constant pain. Central sensitization means something a little different among physicians. Some use the term because a patient reports excess pain due to a minor (e.g., stubbed toe) injury. Other physicians use the term if an expected opioid dosage fails to relieves pain.

IP develops due to one of two pathologic occurrences: (1) nerve injury with bioelectrical blockage, (2) inflammation with tissue destruction. Inflammatory tissue destruction tends to develop down deep or burning type pain sensations. Nerve injury causes a back-up of bioelectricity because the nerve can't pass it. This situation causes great pain on touch, as well as stabbing pain often accompanied by tremors, jerks, and spasms. For example, adhesive arachnoiditis entraps spinal canal nerve roots (cauda equina) in an inflammatory, adhesive mass. The unfortunate person will experience both inflammatory, burning pain as well as stabbing pains as the backed-up bioelectricity detours around the blockage in spurts.

Recognition of IP is easy once someone knows that pain is constant and that there are flares or breakthrough episodes. Pain may often be "burning" or associated with jerks and tremors.

Complications of IP

IP has numerous, severe complications which can shorten life and incapacitate an individual. Totally untreated IP will cause death within days to weeks once it starts. This occurrence, for example, has been observed following injuries to soldiers who could not obtain morphine or other potent pain relievers. Death with IP is due to either heart stoppage (asystole) or adrenal failure. IP is perhaps the most stressful entity that may affect the human body. From the day IP begins, cardiovascular complications will be evident. The key to recognizing IP is a person with constant pain, a history of prior traumatic injury or inflammatory disease, and episodes of tachycardia (elevated pulse rate) and hypertension. IP causes most of its pathologic complications by over-stimulating the cardiovascular, endocrine (hormone), and metabolic-immunologic systems.

It may cause any of the following CV complications:

High blood pressure (hypertension)
Elevated pulse rate (tachycardia)
Arteriosclerosis
Congestive heart failure
Angina pectoris
Myocardial infarction (Heart attack)
Cardiac arrythmias
Sudden CV death (Asystole)

IP causes the pituitary-adrenal-gonadal axis to over-stimulate. The result initially is an excessive release of cortisol and adrenaline from the adrenals. Since IP is constant, the continuous elevation of these hormones leads to alterations in blood glucose and lipids. Persons with IP may show a diabetic or prediabetic profile. Lipids (e.g., cholesterol) may elevate. The pituitary, adrenals, and gonads put out high hormone levels due to the constant stress of IP. These glands may hypertrophy and show as tumors on x-ray. Failure to recognize this development has even led to unnecessary and dangerous surgical removal of pituitary and adrenal glands. In the late stages of IP, however, the glands can't keep up with the stress and demands of IP. Blood levels of cortisol and these other hormones may also drop: pregnenolone, estradiol, dehydroepiandrosterone (DHEA), and testosterone. Cortisol levels may drop so low that Addison's disease is in effect.

Cortisol has been known to drop to such a low level in IP as to cause death. Low levels of other hormones cause a wide variety of pathologic issues included is impaired immunity, fatigue, depression, and mental incapacities.

IP's rise in cortisol followed by exhaustion of testosterone and other hormones has a dramatic, deteriorating effect on bones and teeth. Low hormone level causes calcium to dissolve and leave the teeth, joints, and spine. Vertebrae may become so fragile with osteoporosis that the spine may collapse in places. When calcium leaves the joints, you get arthritis. Don't be surprised if you bite hard on even simi-hard food and have a tooth fall out. Dental decay is usually severe in IP. Osteoporosis of hips and knees makes them so fragile that persons with IP frequently have fractured hips, and arthritic knees.

The impairment of the immune system encourages infections of all kinds as well as reactivation of latent viruses, particularly Epstein Barr Virus (EBV).

The CNS dysfunction of IP leads to what is called dysautonomia. Autonomic means involuntary. A part of the nervous system called autonomic because it functions on its own with no conscious effort by the individual. Much of the autonomic function of the body is through the vagus nerves and what are called adrenergic receptors. Physiologic, autonomic functions include regulation of blood pressure, pulse rate, blood flow, gastrointestinal digestion, skin temperature, and breathing rate.

A key characteristic of the dysautonomia of IP that helps recognize the presence of IP is cold hands and feet. This finding is almost always present in persons with IP. Sometimes the hands turn blue. This is often called Raynaud's phenomenon, as it was named after the physician who discovered it. Dysautonomia may produce sudden hypotension with fainting and bloating, and pain in the intestine. Episodes of diarrhea alternating with constipation may ensue. A diagnosis of irritable bowel syndrome is commonly ascribed to IP patients.

Dysautonomia has led to a concept known as "descending pain." Tissue damage in the brain causes abnormal bioelectric conduction. This may lead to pain signals that descend down the vagus nerve and spinal cord. While this phenomenon is incompletely understood, agents such as tizanidine and clonidine relieve it by activating the adrenergic receptors that control the autonomic nervous system.

The large number and severity of IP complications is largely unknown in both medical and lay circles. These complications and the shortened lifespan they induce have recently caused some states to pass "IP laws" and the California State Medical Board has exempted persons with IP from controlled substance guidelines. Wikipedia notes that IP is often called a "disease" in part due to its serious complications. The complications of IP make it easy to recognize the presence of the condition. It is simply a person with constant pain, who has a history of past trauma or an inflammatory disorder, elevated pulse or blood pressure, and cold hands and feet.

IP is Treated with a Three Component Protocol

IP is a serious, catastrophic condition. Treatment of it is done with a three-component protocol. There is no single drug, exercise, or surgery that will control IP. Below are listed the three essential components of IP treatment. All three are equally critical to long-term care. Medical practitioners have many options for each component.

Component 1: Suppress Inflammation and Autoimmunity

Most IP patients have inflammation both in the CNS and in some muscles, nerves, or joints. Both types of inflammation will have to be treated or it will progressively damage more and more tissue. Inflammation may be generated by autoimmunity from a chronic viral infection. A number of anti-inflammation and autoimmune suppressing agents may be effective. Here are some popular medicinals: ketorolac, methylprednisolone, dexamethasone, whole adrenal gland, curcumin, indomethacin, diclofenac, luteolin, serrapeptase, colchicine.

Component 2: Restoration of Damaged Tissue

There must be a continuous effort to restore damaged tissue since inflammation is persistently damaging tissue. Restoration requires protein/collagen supplements along with vitamins and minerals known to enhance healing. A high protein, anti-inflammatory diet is recommended and described in a later chapter.

We recommend that colostrum and polypeptides be initiated in new IP patients. Colostrum contains a number of restorative hormones. Polypeptides are chains of amino acids. Most IP patients report less pain and greater mobility with colostrum and one or more peptides. Both are non-prescription natural medicinals which have few serious side effects.

Hormone testing for pregnenolone, dehydroepiandrosterone (DHEA), estradiol, and testosterone are recommended. Replenishment of any that are deficient is advised because these hormones all provide some tissue restoration. It is well understood that some laboratory tests are financially prohibitive. In these cases, short hormone trials are warranted. Three hormones with anabolic properties are recommended: human chorionic gonadotropin (HCG), human growth hormone (HGH), and nandrolone.

Electromedical treatment is worthy of clinical trials. Both electric current and electromagnetic administration seem to help individual patients.

Some physical measures help restore neurologic function and reduce pain. They are described in the self-help section of this handbook.

Component 3: Pain Relief

Enough pain control is necessary to carry out activities of daily living and perform normal mental and physical functions without sedation. It is emphasized that pain control is primarily symptomatic and does not prevent deterioration and worsening of the causative, pathologic conditions that underly IP. Pain control by itself cannot substitute or leave off protocol components one and two.

We recommend that new IP patients be started on low dose naltrexone (LDN) and palmitoylethanolamide (PEA). The latter is a newly discovered fatty acid pain reliever and anti-inflammatory that is naturally made in the human body. PEA can be used simultaneously with LDN or by itself for flares. PEA is now being combined with luteolin and other natural or herbal ingredients to be more effective.

Persons with IP will almost always require an agent that enhances or substitutes for gamma aminobutyric acid (GABA). The most popular are gabapentin, pregabalin, and benzodiazepines. The non-opioid pain relievers, ketamine, and oxytocin, are recommended as adjutants to LDN. Kratom and cannabis products (CBD) have become popular. They are legal and readily available in some states. Medicinals that enhance or substitute for dopamine and serotonin may promote pain relief. A list of possible add-on medications is found in a later chapter.

If the above medicinals fail to relieve pain, opioids can be started. One of the weak opioids should be the first prescribed: tramadol, codeine compound, or buprenorphine.

Although more potent opioids have been standard treatment in the past, few new IP patients require them, especially if they are on the 3-component medical protocol. Those persons who are often called “legacy” patients and who have long been on strong opioids often time, for several years. If they function well, they should remain on them with little or no change in dosage. Legacy patients should be warned that they will likely deteriorate unless they initiate suppression of inflammation and restore damaged tissues.

In contrast to the past (this handbook is written in late 2023) long-acting opioids, implanted electrical stimulators, and intrathecal opioids are no longer recommended except after specific clinical trials have been tried and failed to control pain. Trials to be specifically attempted include LDN and/or low dose opioids.

Also, a potent short-acting opioid such as hydrocodone, hydromorphone, morphine, oxycodone, or fentanyl dermal patch with injectable hydromorphone for flares or breakthrough pain, should be attempted before long-acting opioids or an invasive implant is attempted.

Long acting and intrathecal opioids should only be started for end-of-life care because they suppress the endocrine system and may even cause a hyperalgesic state that renders all opioids ineffective. As stated above, however, some unusual IP patients have long-tolerated and function well with long-acting and intrathecal opioids.

Tapering or reduction of opioids and other medications should not be done in a bonafide IP patient unless the patient requests it be done. IP is such a serious disease that it is always palliative and will produce a premature death if medication is reduced without a specific patient request and plan to restart if pain and withdrawal symptoms emerge. IP, by definition, is a severe pain that is incurable and has life-shortening complications. Recognition and documentation of IP is essential since care is lifelong and not subject to significant medication reduction once a regimen is found to be effective.

Nerve Damage and Bioelectricity in IP

All persons with IP initiate the pathologic process that leads to their condition with trauma or an inflammatory disease. Trauma includes a fall, medical procedures, and physical alterations. Trauma that causes IP usually involves the head, spinal cord, or spine including the intervertebral discs. The traumatic events that lead to IP initially produce nerve damage. The nerves may be microscopic as in the brain and spinal canal or large as in the chest wall, joint, or extremity.

Proper treatment of IP requires knowledge of how bioelectricity is conducted in nerves. Bioelectrical nerve conduction takes place in all tissues and organs of the body including the brain, spinal cord, muscles, heart, and extremities. It is often evaluated by electrocardiogram, electromyogram, and other devices that assesses flow of bioelectricity in nerves.

Impaired conduction or flow of bioelectricity in A nerve occurs when the injury or damage causes a tissue blockage with a tear, scar, or compression. The body's bioelectricity travels at a normal speed and intensity. If bioelectricity is interrupted or blocked it backs up which may result in dull, agonizing, or burning pain. Backed up or retained bioelectricity will accumulate to a point where it eventually has to "jump" over the blockage or takes a detour around it. Blocked or retained bioelectricity pain may be accompanied by stabbing, tremors, shakes, or jerks since it tends to escape the blockage in spurts. A condition called "restless leg" may result.

Unfortunately, backed up or blocked bioelectricity is hot and destructive to tissue. In effect, it fries tissue like meat in a hot pan on the stove. When a tissue is burnt and hot it is said to be "inflamed." The tissue becomes painful, and it may be permanently destroyed. This message is critical. A nerve injury or blockage causes a vicious cycle:

Damaged Nerve

↓

Bioelectricity Blockage

↓

Inflammation

↓

More Nerve Damage

↓

More Pain

Treatment and control measures which attempted to ameliorate nerve damage and blocked bioelectricity date far back in time. Most were discovered by ancient people out of sheer desperation. Some measures still have merit today.

Basically, these remedies "pull out" or enhance bioelectric conduction. These ancient remedies include copper jewelry and magnets. Water soaking, massage, and application of heat all have merit. Acupuncture and needle insertion are therapeutic since the metal in the needle, usually stainless steel made from iron, has a positive electric charge which attracts bioelectricity that has a negative charge. This alleviates pain by pulling out the "charge."

For obvious reasons, many medical practitioners like to call the pain of impaired bioelectric conduction, neuropathic pain. Also, physicians have started calling pharmacological medicines, that improve bioelectric conduction, neuropathic agents. These agents enhance or substitute for the neurotransmitters, gamma amino butyric acid (GABA) which conducts bioelectricity. Popular neuropathic agents include gabapentin, pregabalin, (Lyrica®), baclofen, and the class of drugs known as benzodiazepines.

Inflammation and Autoimmunity: New Discoveries

For literally centuries, physicians have assumed that nerve damage was the sole, underlying cause of IP. In recent years, however, multiple discoveries have revealed that IP is the result of inflammation as well as nerve damage. There are two inflammatory components in IP: (1) inflammation in tissues outside the CNS, and (2) inflammation inside the CNS (called neuroinflammation).

An inflammatory disorder or process outside the CNS is almost always a contributor to the pathologic sequence of events that leads to IP. The majority of today's IP cases we review have usually started with one of three events. Genetic connective tissue disease, especially EDS, may develop areas of inflammation in various bodily tissues due to a collagen defect in connective tissue. Microtears occur which lead to inflammation. Traumatic nerve injury leads to bioelectric retention which causes inflammation. A third inflammatory situation may develop without an apparent genetic disease or injury.

These persons develop an inflammatory disease such as fibromyalgia or thyroiditis without any obvious facilitating event.

Interestingly, most persons who develop IP report that they have experienced multiple inflammatory conditions before they developed IP. The attached Table lists many of the inflammatory conditions that pre-date IP.

At some time after a traumatic injury or inflammatory disorder occurs, constant pain develops. As stated in a former chapter, glial and microglial cells in the CNS activate, produce inflammation, and generate constant pain. IP is, in actuality, the entity that results from a pathologic process that begins with an inflammatory condition outside the CNS.

A recent discovery is that some viruses which were originally thought to be harmless and live in the human body as parasites may actually activate at times and produce inflammation. The main virus that does this is called Epstein-Barr. It is named after the two scientists who discovered this virus in tumors called lymphomas (hereafter EBV). Although EBV is the main virus implicated in IP, other viruses and Lyme infection, which is a bacteria, may potentiate or accentuate EBV. To date, cytomegalovirus, herpes six, and covid have been reported to partner or enhance the adverse effects of EBV.

Viral invasion and autoimmunity appear to be logical facilitators of IP. An inflammatory condition may initiates a pathologic sequence that ends with CNS neuroinflammation and IP.

COMMON INFLAMMATORY CONDITIONS THAT PRE-DATE IP	
1	Arthritis
2	Burning mouth or feet
3	Carpal tunnel
4	Chiari conditions
5	Dry eyes (Sjogren's)
6	Fibromyalgia
7	Food-medicine sensitivities
8	Hashimoto's thyroiditis
9	Herniated/slipped discs
10	Herpes
11	Spinal canal cysts (Tarlov's)
12	Irritable bowel
13	Mast cell activation (hives/welts)
14	Migraine
15	Small fiber neuropathy
16	Psoriasis
17	Shingles
18	Spinal fluid leaks
19	Temporal mandibular joint (TMJ)

The presence of one or more of these inflammatory conditions usually pre-date the development of IP. The Epstein Barr Virus

(EBV) may facilitate the development of these conditions by autoimmunity and/or tissue invasion.

The Critical Neurotransmitter-Receptor Systems

A pain relief drug, whether it be natural, herbal, or synthetic, activates or triggers action sites in the CNS called receptors. These sites are called receptors because they "receive" a triggering biochemical called a neurotransmitter. To date, seven neurotransmitter-receptor systems have been identified that may relieve pain. We believe that persons with IP must activate or stimulate at least two of these systems in order to relieve pain. A medicinal that relieves pain must either enhance replace or substitute for a neurotransmitter. The most dominant receptor for pain relief is the endorphin receptor, and the second most critical is called the gamma aminobutyric acid (GABA) receptor. Most IP patients recognize the critical importance of these two receptors since they have found relief with an endorphin substitute or enhance such as an opioid or a GABA substitute or enhances such as gabapentin (Neurontin®), pregabalin (Lyrica®), diazepam (Valium®), or carisoprodol (Soma®).

Most IP patients may also need to activate some of the other neurotransmitter-receptor systems, to attain some relief. At this time, there is no test to determine which systems need to be activated. Only a clinical trial with medication will determine which neurotransmitter-receptor systems will provide pain relief.

Shown here are the seven neurotransmitter-receptor systems and some of the common medicinals that are used to activate them. Also shown here are single amino acids that make some of the neurotransmitters. Amino acids are often called precursors of a neurotransmitter.

TABLE

	Amino Acid Precursor	Neurotransmitter
1	Phenylalanine/tyrosine	Dopamine
2	Tryptophan	Serotonin
3	Glutamine	Gamma aminobutyric acid (GABA)

The neurotransmitters in the table are made from singular amino acids. Some IP patients achieve pain relief by taking the amino acid precursor.

TABLE

Neurotransmitter-Receptor Systems that Control and Relieve Pain

MAJOR

Endorphin
opioids, oxytocin
naltrexone, kratom

GABA
gabapentin, Lyrica®
Soma®, Valium®, Xanax®

SECONDARY

Dopamine/Noradrenaline
Adderall®, phentermine
methylphenidate,
dextroamphetamine

Serotonin
Zoloft®, Cymbalta®
nortriptyline
amitriptyline

Cannabinoid
CBD
marijuana

N-Methyl-d-Aspartate (NMDA)
ketamine
dextromethorphan

Adrenergic
clonidine
tizanidine

Some of the common medicinals used to activate or enhance each system are shown here.

Unfortunately, CNS inflammation may cripple or damage one or more of the neurotransmitter-receptor systems. Tissue damage to these systems can be visualized on some brain scans and MRI's. The "Knock-out" of these systems is the forerunner of constant pain and its complications. The three-component medical protocol described and recommended in this handbook is targeted in great part at restoring the neurotransmitter-receptor systems.

Self-Help Section

How to Build an Effective IP Program

Treatment and control of IP requires study and diligence to build an effective program. IP has multiple causative factors and complications. No one size fits all. The biggest mistake is to believe that a singular, symptomatic treatment such as an opioid, implanted electrical stimulator, or surgery will solve your problem. This approach may work for a while, but most persons with IP have a progressive disorder that will worsen unless a three-component medical protocol is implemented. There are some sequential steps we recommend to assist in building an effective program, which are described here.

To help you build an effective program, you will need to have a close family member or friend in which you can confide and who will assist you. Don't rely on medical practitioners to do all your care. Study the reasons you have pain and what we know about IP. Don't make plans for some exercise or dietary measure that you won't religiously do <u>EVERY DAY.</u> Be practical.

I recommend you think about it like building a house or a business. Take one step at a time. Keep what works but keep trying new ideas and measures. The following chapters are sequential building blocks. Even if you already have a good program, review the steps here. Chances are you'll pick up a tip or two to enhance your current program.

Step One: Document Your IP and Its Cause

You wouldn't likely be reading this handbook unless you have IP or are a family member of one who does have it. In today's health system, you may not get much help, and you might even be insulted, humiliated, or condemned if you tell someone you are a "pain patient." Lots of emergency rooms, hospitals, health plans, and practitioners don't want you around.

If you are not sure you have IP, review the former chapters in this handbook. Make a written record of the date when you had your initiating trauma or inflammatory disorder. List what your symptoms and treatments have been since your inciting event. Record your IP complications. In particular, document your blood pressure, pulse rate, laboratory tests, and magnetic resonance imaging (MRI) studies that relate to your case. Make a written medical record that you can carry with you to your medical visits.

Always refer to your condition as to the major cause of your IP and not just IP. For example, you may find that you will get better care if you refer to yourself as an "arachnoiditis" or "stroke" patient rather than an IP patient. It may be unfair and callous, but many parties have great bias against pain patients.

IP is an uncommon condition. Few persons in the medical system have ever heard of IP, so you must not only have a written, transportable record, but be ready and able to explain and educate about IP to any concerned party. Be able to always explain your basic cause and inciting event.

Step Two: Keep What Works

Make an inventory of everything you have tried to control your IP. This not only includes medications but exercises, dietary measures, and social activities. Continue anything that works even a little. Then start building your three-component program.

Think back. Did you try something many months or years ago that helped you? If so, restart it. Have you been taking a drug or exercise that hasn't helped? Throw those away.

Be practical. Don't kid yourself. Do only dietary, physical, and medical measures you will do every day. IP needs daily care and not just something you do once in a while or when you get "around to it."

What about your supplies? Do you have a local pharmacy, health food store, and internet site that have been helpful? Don't change just for the sake of changing. Stick with what works. Start building a program now and continually try to upgrade it.

Step Three: Do You Have Ehlers-Danlos Syndrome?

Amazingly, many persons who develop IP in their middle or older ages realize they have a genetic-inherited disease that may be the basic cause of their IP. These genetic diseases develop a variety of inflammatory disorders that may lead to IP. Also, any traumatic injury may have a more damaging result than in other persons. The three most common are: (1) Ehlers-Danlos Syndrome, (2) ankylosing spondylitis, (3) scoliosis. There are also some very rare genetic-inherited diseases (e.g., hydrocephalus, Marfan, porphyria, or others) that may lead to IP.

Most persons are well aware if they have scoliosis. Ankylosing spondylitis is a painful, inflammatory, fibrotic disease of the spine. It is diagnosed with a blood test for an antigen called HCA-B27. Any person with a chronically painful spine should have this test.

The most common genetic-inherited disease that leads to IP is a connective tissue disorder called Ehlers-Danlos Syndrome (EDS. This disorder is a defect in the production the collagen in connecting tissue that supports bodily structures and organs. The defect in collagen causes microscopic tears and the development of inflammation and pain. This especially affects intervertebral discs, linings of blood vessels, spinal canal cover, joints, and small nerve fibers. Weakened tissues due to inadequate collagen is "fertile ground" for the invasion of opportunistic parasites like EBV. It is critical that every person with IP determine if they have EDS. A screening test for EDS is provided. If you score high on this test you will need to consult a medical practitioner who will do what is called a Breighton Score and possibly some genetic tests to validate the presence of EDS. Also, you will need to begin an aggressive program to restore and strengthen defective tissue. A failure to recognize and deal with EDS makes it difficult to control IP.

Screening Test for Ehlers-Danlos Syndrome (EDS)

	QUESTION	Yes	No
1	Do you have pain in multiple locations?		
2	Do you have extreme fatigue?		
3	Are you clumsy sometimes and fall or walk into objects?		
4	Are some of the joints in your hands, feet, elbow, hips, or knees "loose" or quite flexible?		
5	Have you had a lot of sprains or joint dislocations?		
6	Is your skin thin in places?		
7	Are you double-jointed or able to bend your fingers, arms, or ankle backwards?		
8	Are your hands and feet cold much of the time?		
9	Do you bruise easily or have bruises that suddenly occur?		
10	Is your skin "stretchy" in some places?		
11	Are you constipated a lot?		
12	Do you suffer from "heartburn" or frequent episodes of food regurgitation?		

If you answer yes to 6 or more of the 12 you likely have "Ehlers-Danlos Syndrome" and are at high risk of developing complications of adhesive arachnoiditis and other causes of IP. Please inform your medical practitioners of the results of this test.

Step Four: Screen for the Common Causes of IP

Many persons with IP have never been given a specific diagnosis or they have been given a non-specific one such as neuropathy, central pain, arthritis, failed back, or degenerative pain. The two most common causes of IP today are adhesive arachnoiditis (AA) and complex regional pain syndrome (CRPS). Both of these conditions require some specific therapeutic measures, so it is essential to know if you have either or both. Take the screening tests offered here and relay the results to your family and medical practitioners.

SCREENING TEST FOR LUMBAR-SACRAL ADHESIVE ARACHNOIDITIS		**Yes**	**No**
	QUESTIONS		
1	In addition to chronic pain, do you ever experience sharp, stabbing pains in your lower back when you twist, turn or bend?		
2	Do you ever experience bizarre skin sensations such as crawling insects or water dripping down one or both legs?		
3	Do you ever have burning, tingling, or a sensation of walking on broken glass in your feet and/or toes?		
4	Does your pain lessen when you stand or recline?		
5	Do you have leg weakness and/or pain that radiates down one or both legs?		
6	Do you experience any bladder dysfunction such as dribbling, or difficulty when starting or stopping urination?		
7	Do you sometimes have a headache along with blurred vision?		

If you answer yes to four or more of these seven questions, in the above table, you most likely have AA.

SCREENING TEST FOR COMPLEX REGIONAL PAIN SYNDROME (CRPS)			
	QUESTIONS	**Yes**	**No**
1	Do you have burning pain?		
2	Do you have increased skin sensitivity to touch?		
3	Have you had changes in skin temperature in an area compared to other areas?		
4	Has your skin changed color becoming blotchy, purple, pale, or red?		
5	Has your skin texture changed in areas becoming shiny or thin, or excessively sweaty?		
6	Have you experienced changes in nail or hair growth patterns in painful areas?		
7	Do you have swelling and stiffness in the affected joints?		
8	Do you have difficulty walking because of stiffness and decreased ability to move the affected body part?		
9	Are your symptoms asymmetrical, on one side but not the other?		
10	Is your pain greater than usual for the type of injury you have?		
11	Is the painful limb or area swollen and the skin shiny?		

12	Do you have bone changes in the affected area?		

If you answer yes to eight or more of these twelve questions, you most likely have "Complex Regional Pain Syndrome."

Step Five: Start the Intractable Pain Diet

IP is an uncommon disorder, and it requires an uncommon diet. Unfortunately, the hormonal changes produced by IP may leave one with little appetite except for an intense craving for sugars and starches. The IP diet consists of certain "must eat" categories of food. A technical name for the diet is "High Protein, Anti-inflammatory."

Protein: It provides the amino acid building blocks that are necessary for production of most neurotransmitters that relieve pain. They also help restore and build damaged tissues.

You must eat one or more of these high protein foods each day: fish, chicken, turkey, beef, pork, eggs, cottage cheese, shrimp.

Spirulina, algae, black beans, and pumpkin seeds have a fairly high protein content. If you can't or won't eat any of these, you must obtain protein powder drinks and/or protein bars from A health food store. Whey and soy are acceptable.

Vegetables and Fruits: These vegetables and fruits have anti-inflammatory activity. You must eat one or more each day: carrot, broccoli, radish, blueberry, apple, celery, brussel sprouts, onion, blackberry, beets, spinach, lettuce, raspberry, tomatoes, cucumbers, watermelon, strawberry.

Drinks: The following drinks are acceptable: coffee, tea, diet soda, water, occasional alcohol! Sugar in drinks (labeled as carbohydrates) should not be consumed.

Restrict these foods to Control Weight and lower Blood Glucose Levels: milk, regular soda, fruit juice, bread, rolls, buns, pies, cakes, pizza.

Daily Supplements: amino acid blend (powder, capsules, drink) and/or collagen. A Multivitamin-mineral tab or capsule is recommended.

Step Six: Start Prophylaxis of Ebstein Barr Virus

Over 90% of the world's population carries EBV as a latent (silent or quiet) parasitic infection in their body. Most persons contract EBV in infancy, and the parasite remains quiet, silent, and harmless in the body's lymphocytes throughout life in most cases. Sometimes EBV activates when a person is in their teenage or young adult years The condition is known as "infectious mononucleosis."

Recent scientific studies show that EBV may periodically activate and cause a variety of pathologic conditions including some cancers, multiple sclerosis, and rheumatoid arthritis. It may periodically reactivate and cause inflammation in multiple tissues that lead to or aggravate IP. EBV especially aggravates or possibly initiates adhesive arachnoiditis, complex regional pain syndrome, and multiple herniated discs.

EBV may reactivate during times of stress including severe pain, trauma, infections, or emotional distress. It is recommended that every person with IP test for the EBV antibodies (IgG- not IgM) that indicate if there has been periodic reactivation of EBV in the past or present.

<u>Blood Testing for Reactivation:</u> EBV antibody testing is an indicator of both past and current reactivity. Three tests of IgG (not IgM) antibodies are recommended:

1. Viral capsule antigen (VCA-IgG), past episodes of reactivation
2. EBV nuclear antigen (EBNA-IgG), past episodes of reactivation
3. EBV early antigen (EA-IgG), current reactivation

If a person with IP shows high levels of EBV IgG antibodies, we recommend one or more of the agents listed in the Table that have been shown in laboratory studies to inhibit EBV reactivation. If a person with IP shows current reactivation with elevated early antigen antibody (EBNA-IgG), a short course of an antiviral agent plus one or more inhibitory agents is recommended.

The purpose of EBV prophylaxis is to keep one's IP condition from progressing due to EBV reactivation.

Below are listed inhibitors of EBV reactivation which have been identified in the reference listed here:

Cimetidine
Vitamins A, C, D
Resveratrol
Luteolin
Apigenin
Astralagus
L-arginine
Curcumin

Reference: Kerr JR. Epstein Barr virus (EBV) reactivation and therapeutic inhibitors. J Clin Path 2019; 0:1-8.

In addition to the above, some other prophylactic agents have become popular. Perhaps the most popular is monolaurin which is an ingredient of coconut oil. Selenium, magnesium, vitamin B-12, and K2, have also become popular. At this time there are no controlled studies to assess prophylaxis, effectiveness, but our clinical observations suggest that prophylaxis is effective, since patients have clinically improved often taking one or more of the recommended inhibitors. Consequently, we highly recommend that one or more EBV inhibitors be used to hopefully prevent IP from progressing.

Step Seven: Start An Herbal Anti-inflammatory Agent

If you have constant pain, it means you have inflammation (called neuroinflammation) in your CNS. You likely have one or more other inflammatory conditions, such as fibromyalgia, thyroiditis, or carpal tunnel syndrome. To achieve some relief and recovery from IP, it is essential that you take one or more anti-inflammatory agents. Many persons with IP have been led to believe that symptomatic pain treatment with opioids, electrical stimulators, or other pain relief medication is all you need. Nothing could be more erroneous. If the inflammation that causes IP isn't suppressed and hopefully eliminated, IP will eventually worsen at which time a bed-bound state and early death will occur.

Ideally a person with IP should have these blood tests for inflammatory markers to see how severe their inflammation may be. If any of these markers are elevated it is essential to increase one's intake of anti-inflammatory agents.

Inflammation Markers

C-reactive protein (CRP)
Erythrocyte sedimentation rate (ESR)
White blood cell count
Cytokine panel of interleukins

Unfortunately, blood tests for inflammatory markers are expensive, so physicians may not be able to order the tests since health plans won't pay for them. Even if tests cannot be obtained, a person with IP must go ahead and begin treatment with one or more of the herbal agents listed in the attached table.

Why herbal agents? Most prescription anti-inflammatory agents are made for short-term usage in the treatment of an acute medical problem. Most IP patients can't tolerate long-term use of most anti-inflammatory agents. IP is a lifetime condition, so natural, or herbal agents are preferentially recommended to suppress inflammation. They have few side effects and cross the blood brain barrier to enter the spinal fluid. They also seldom adversely react with other medications. Some may prevent EBV reactivation.

TABLE
HERBAL-NATURAL AGENTS FOR IP

Turmeric/curcumin
Serrapeptase
Desiccated adrenal
Traumeel
Luteolin
Astragalus

The anti-inflammatory agents listed here can be rotated and more than one can be taken in a single day. Dosage instructions are on the label. Persons with IP will usually need one and a half or two times the labeled dosage. All agents listed here are non-prescription and readily available, inexpensive and can be purchased from multiple sources.

If inflammation persists despite the use of natural or herbal agents as determined by blood tests, the use of corticosteroids, ketorolac, or other prescription agents will be necessary.

Step Eight: Special Physical Measures for IP

IP requires some special physical measures to keep it from progressing. Physical measures are not primarily done to build strength, physical appearance, lose weight, or improve cardiovascular output. They have these purposes: (1) improve spinal fluid flow, (2) remove excess bioelectricity and inflammatory toxins.

Blockage of bioelectricity due to damaged nerves and the accumulation of inflammatory toxins will cause IP to progressively worsen. Even though severe pain will naturally keep your mind focused on the pain, you must force yourself to do some of the physical measures listed here. You can actually do some of the measures if you are bed bound. What's more, some of the measures listed here may provide some short-term pain relief, although the main purpose is to stop disease progression and obtain some long-term relief and recovery. Review the measures shown here and pick ones that you will do EVERY DAY. There are some that you may want to do multiple times a day.

Purpose: Increase Lymph and Spinal Fluid Flow

- Rocking chair or swing
- Gentle bouncing (rebounding) on a trampoline
- Deep breathing. Take in oxygen to your maximum. Hold it for five seconds and exhale slowly through pursed lips.
- Walk with arm swings. If unable to walk, you can stand or even recline and swing your arms. Do this several times a day. Daily walks with arm swings are optimal if you are physically able.
- Apply heat with an old-fashioned water bottle or heating pad to painful areas.

Purpose: Extract Excess Bioelectricity and Inflammatory Toxins

- Water soak in a Jacuzzi, swimming pool, or bathtub for 10 to 15 minutes a day. If not available, warm showers will do. Do one to two times a day.

- Soak feet in Epsom Salts or an herbal concoction.
- Rub painful areas with a magnet for only a few seconds and do this multiple times a day.
- Wear a copper bracelet or anklet.
- Stretch and flex your neck, ankles, arms, and legs. Do multiple times a day. You can do this standing, sitting, or reclining.

We also support light weightlifting, treadmill walking, or stationary bicycle riding if one is physically capable. Do not over-exert or cause pain or fatigue.

Step Nine: Build a Sleep Program

Adequate sleep is critical to control IP because the body makes many of its pain control neurotransmitters and hormones during sleep. Most persons with constant pain have to take a sleep assist medication to attain some sleep.

Be prepared to be able to sleep for only two to four hours at a stretch. You may awaken during the night. Don't be concerned about short stretches of sleep. Try to get a total of about six to eight hours of sleep in a 24-hour period.

If you currently take a sleep medication that works for you, continue it. When it comes to IP, there is no good or bad sleep medication – take what works. The only caveat is that you don't want a sleep medication to make you sleepy or groggy during the following day.

If you have chronic insomnia and have no prescription medication to assist you, I recommend the following which you can obtain from your local pharmacy or health food store.

1. Diphenhydramine (Benadryl®, 25 mg) plus
2. Tryptophan (500 to 1000 mg)

Option: Add melatonin 5 to 10 mg.

Medical marijuana and cannabis products have become popular sleep aids. These are acceptable if they don't make you sleepy or groggy the next day.

Tryptophan is recommended to take with whatever medication you take for sleep. Why? It is the precursor of serotonin which is one of the CNS neurotransmitters that relieves pain. Our general experience is that IP patients achieve about 10-20 per cent more pain relief the day following the use of tryptophan at bedtime.

The antidepressant drugs, amitriptyline and nortriptyline have been favorite sleep aids for pain patients for many years. This is because they activate the serotonin and possibly other neurotransmitter-receptor systems in the CNS. Most medical practitioners will prescribe these older drugs on request since they have proved to be inexpensive, effective, and safe for the vast majority of pain patients.

Step Ten: Start a Tissue Restoration Program

IP with its constant pain indicates you probably have an ongoing inflammatory-autoimmune process that is progressively destroying your nerve tissue and making you worse. Even though pain relief is obviously at the top of your needs and desires, you must start a tissue restoration program to combat the persistent assault and degeneration of your nerves by inflammation.

Be clearly advised. In days gone by, there was the false belief that nerve tissue could not be regenerated or restored. We now clearly know that almost all damaged bodily tissues including muscle, fascia, and nerves can all regenerate and be restored to a great extent. Cure or near cure of all conditions that lead to IP depend on restoration of damaged tissue.

My first two tissue restoration recommendations are: (1) daily supplement with collagen or a blend of amino acids, (2) colostrum supplementation. This medicinal is the milky hormone produced by female mammals, including humans, immediately after giving birth. It contains multiple hormones and anti-infectious agents. The natural purpose of colostrum is to promote tissue growth and protect against infections. Not only does a newborn baby benefit from colostrum, so does a person with IP. Colostrum is available from several vendors. Get started with it. Follow the instructions on the label. No prescription is needed.

Once you are started with collagen or amino acids, and colostrum, consider starting any of the below-listed measures. You probably can't overdo it. Pick and choose from these options:

- Medical Agents
    - ✓ Peptides
    - ✓ Desiccated adrenal
    - ✓ Dehydroepiandrosterone (DHEA)
- Electromedical Administration
    - ✓ Microcurrent
    - ✓ Multicurrent
    - ✓ Electromagnetic

There are potent anabolic (tissue restoration) hormones that are relatively new in the treatment of IP. They include human chorionic gonadotropin (HCG) and nandrolone. These hormones can only be prescribed by a licensed medical practitioner. They should be considered as a trial once a three-component protocol is in place.

Step Eleven: Start Natural Pain Relief and See Your Doctor

To control IP and obtain some relief and recovery, a person with IP must usually build a program of both natural-herbal pain relievers as well as prescription pain relievers which must be prescribed by a licensed medical professional. Persons with IP must assume they will require pain relievers for life. Unfortunately, however, many different parties in society have control over the availability of prescription pain relievers. Steady, predictable availability of supplies is not possible.

The focus in this handbook is on the two major neurotransmitter-receptor systems that relieve IP: (1) endorphin, (2) gamma aminobutyric acid (GABA).

In recent years, a small number of non-prescription, natural-herbal pain relievers have been identified that enhance or substitute for endorphin and GABA. You must learn these. Some IP patients start treating their IP in its early or mild stage with only natural or herbal medicinals, and they satisfactorily manage their pain. Others can minimize their need for prescription pain relievers. The simultaneous use of both natural-herbal pain relievers and prescription pain relievers will usually provide the best pain relief.

Our recommendation is to select a natural-herbal medicinal from each of the two major classes listed below. Try it for a few days. If it doesn't help, switch to another. Keep searching to find one or more that help so you don't have to totally rely on prescription pain relievers.

Once you have gone through the steps listed in this handbook, it is time to consult your medical practitioner. Most are willing and knowledgeable enough to assist with at least some pain and anti-inflammation relief. Hopefully, your medical practitioner will help with the entire three component protocol required for treatment of IP.

If you attend a pain clinic, you may find that they aren't too interested in providing three component care. Due to a number of factors, they may only focus on addiction treatment or invasive medical procedures.

TABLE

Some Non-prescription, Natural, or Herbal Pain Relievers

Endorphin System	GABA System
Peptides	Kava
Kratom	Ashwagandha
Opium poppy seeds	Valerian root
Akua manna	
Agmatine	

Once you have gone through the steps in this handbook, consult your doctor. Take your written medical record to your doctor including laboratory tests and x-rays. The more information about your IP condition that you can provide your doctor, the more help he/she can provide.

Summary

There is a subgroup of persons with chronic pain who develop biologic changes in the CNS that cause constant, unrelenting, debilitating pain and suffering. This condition is now referred to as IP. The constancy of the pain is a profound stress on bodily functions, so a myriad of cardiovascular, endocrine, metabolic, immunologic, and gastrointestinal complications will occur. Lack of or undertreatment of IP will result in a shortened lifespan.

Persons with IP who achieve the best pain relief and quality of life follow most of the steps listed in this handbook. They also join IP support groups and stay informed on the latest research and discoveries.

IP is poorly recognized and treated at this time. The intent of this handbook is to assist patients, families, and medical practitioners to recognize and treat this uncommon malady with a three-component protocol.

Glossary of Terms

Adhesive Arachnoiditis: An intraspinal canal inflammatory disorder in which there is a clump or mass of cauda equina nerve roots that are glued by adhesions to the arachnoid-dural covering of the spinal canal.

Autoimmunity: A disease process that occurs due to some element or toxin in the body that attacks and destroys tissue.

Bioelectricity: The electricity formed in tissue that fosters muscular movement and neurologic function.

Chronic Pain: A pain that persists longer than the usual healing time of about ninety days.

Connective Tissue Disorder: A genetic disease in which collagen in tissue is deficient or weak so tissues subsequently develops inflammation and pain.

Corticoid or Corticosteroid: A pharmaceutical that is chemically related to cortisone.

Ehlers-Danlos Syndrome: A genetic-connective tissue disorder named after two physicians who first described the condition.

Epstein Barr Virus: A virus in the herpes class that is a normal human parasite but may activate and produce a number of pathologic conditions. Named after the scientists who discovered the virus in a cancer.

Herb: A medicinal that comes from a plant or botanical.

Inflammation: Tissue that is red, hot, and dying.

Intractable Pain: Constant, incurable pain that produces cardiovascular, respiratory, gastrointestinal, endocrine, and metabolic complications.

Latent Phase: A viral state after initial infection when a virus of other infection is quiet, silent, and harmless.

Lytic Phase: Period in which a virus is multiplying by dividing itself by lysis.

Natural: A medicinal that is made in the human body.

Receptor: A molecular site composed of protein which receives a neurotransmitter or biochemical and then creates some function.

References

1. Apkarian AV, Bushnell MC, Treede RD, Zubieta JK. Human brain mechanisms of pain perception and regulation in health and disease. Eur J Pain 2005 9 :463-484.

2. Apkarian AV, Sosa Y, Sont S, et al. Chronic back pain is associated with decreased prefrontal and thalamic gray matter density. J Neurosci 2004; 24:10410-10415.

3. Austin PJ, Moaleno-Taylor G. The neuro-immune balance in neuropathic pain: involvement of inflammatory immune cells, immune-like glial cells and cytokines. J Neuroimmunol 2010; 229:26-50.

4. Bilello J, Tennant F. Patterns of chronic inflammation in extensively treated patients with arachnoiditis and chronic intractable pain. Postgrad Med 2016; 92:1-5.

5. Castori M, Voermann NC. Neurological manifestations of "Ehlers-Danlos Syndromes. Iran J of Neurol 2014; 13:190-208.

6. Cauda F, Palermo S, Costa T, et al. Gray matter alterations in chronic pain: a network-oriented-meta-analytic approach. Neuroimage Clin 2014; 4:676-688.

7. Cohen M, Quintner J, Buchanan D. Is chronic pain a disease? Pain Med 2013; 14:1284-1288.

8. Davis KD. Is chronic pain a disease: Evaluating pain and nociception through self-report and neuroimaging. J Pain 2013; 14:332-333.

9. Glynn CJ, Lloyd JW. Biochemical changes associated with intractable pain. Br Med J 1978; 1:280-281.

10. Harley JB, et al. Transcription factors operate across disease loci, with EBNA2 implicated in autoimmunity. Nat Genet 2018; 50:699-707

11. Harrow T. Epstein-Barr virus could be a cause of multiple autoimmune disorders. VA Research Currents April 18, 2018.

12. Hayashida KJ, Obata H. Strategies to treat chronic pain and strengthen impaired descending noradrenergic inhibitory system. Int J Mol Sci 2019; 20:822-833.

13. Henderson FC, Austin C, Benzel E, et al. Neurological and spinal manifestations of the Ehlers-Danlos Syndromes. Amer J Men Gen 2017;175C195-211.

14. Hung AL, Lim M, Doshi TC. Targeting cytokines for treatment of neuropathic pain. Scand J Pain 2017; 17:287-293.

15. Hunt JH, Linnett MJ. Intractable pain. Brit Med J 1960;(June):1726-1729.

16. Indari O, Tiwari D, Tanwar M, et al. Early biomolecular changes in brain microvascular endothelial cells under Epstein-Barr virus influence: A Raman microspectroscopic investigation. Integr Biol 2022; 14:89-97.

17. Indari O, Jakhomola S, Pathak DK, et al. Comparative account of biomolecular changes post Epstein Barr virus infection of the neuronal and glial cells using Raman microspectroscopy. ACS Chem Neurosci 2022; 13:1627-1637.

18. Jakhmola S, Jha HM. Glial cell response to Epstein Barr Virus infection: a plausible contribution to virus-associated inflammatory reactions in the brain. Virology 2021; 559:182-195.

19. Javida E, Magnus T. Autoimmunity after ischemic stroke and brain injury. Front Immunol 2019; 10:1-12.

20. Kerr J. Epstein Barr Virus (EBV) reactivation and therapeutic inhibitors. J Clin Pathol 2019; 0:1-8.

21. Kiefer, etal. Effects of dexamethasone on microglial activation in vitro. J Neuroimmunology 1991; 34:99-108.

22. Kiguch et al. Chemokines and cytokines in neuroinflammation leading to neuropathic pain. Curr Opinion Pharmacol 2012; 12:55-61.

23. Lei ZM, Rao CV. Neural actions of luteinizing hormone and human chorionic gonadotropin. Seminar Reprod Med 2001; 19:103-109.

24. Loggia MI, Chunde DB, Oluwaseum A, et al. Evidence for brain glial activation in chronic pain patients. Brain 2015; 138:604-615.

25. Martikaineh K, et al. Chronic pain is associated with alterations in dopamine neurotransmission in the ventral striatum. J Neurosci 2015; 35:9957-9965.

26. May A, Boorsok D, Becerra L. Chronic pain may change the structure of the brain. Pain 2008; 137:7–15.

27. Mika J, Zychowska M, Popiolek-Barczy K, et al. Importance of glial activation in neuropathic pain. Eur J Pharmacol 2013; 716:106-119.

28. Millon MJ. Descending control of pain. Prog Neurobiol 2002; 66:355-474.

29. Moltner A, Holz R, Strian F. Heart rate changes as an autonomic component of the pain response. Pain 1990; 43:81-89.

30. Raffaeli W, Arando E. Pain as a disease: an overview. J Pain Res 2017; 10:2003-2008.

31. Sevesto S, Merli P, Ruggier M, et al. Ehlers-Danlos Syndrome and neurological features: a review. Childs Neuro Syst 2011; 27:365-371.

32. Shenkin HA. Effect of pain on diurnal pattern of plasma corticoid levels. Neurology 1964; 14:1112-1115.

33. Takahashi H, Suguro T, Okazima Y, et al. Inflammatory cytokines in the herniated disc of the lumbar spine. Spine 1996; 21:218-224.

34. Takedo, et al. Effect of methylprednisolone on neuropathic pain and spinal glial activation in rats. Anesthesiology 2004; 100:1249-1257.

35. Tennant F. Human chorionic gonadotropin in pain treatment. Prac Pain Manag 2009; 9:25-27.

36. Tennant F, Hermann L. Intractable or chronic pain: there is a difference. West J Med 2000; 173:306.

37. Tennant F, Herman L. Using biologic markers to identify legitimate chronic pain. Amer Clin Lab 2002; 21:14- 18.

38. Tennant F. The physiologic effects of pain on the endocrine system. Pain Ther 2013; 2:75-86.

39. Tsuda M. Microglia in the spinal cord and neuropathic pain. J Diabetes Investig 2016; 7:17-26.

40. Whendon JM, Glassey D. Cerebrospinal fluid stasis and its clinical significance. Altern Ther Health Med 2009; 15:54-60.

41. Zang Y, Chee A, Shi P, et al. Intervertebral disc cells produce interleukins found in patients with back pain. Am J Phys Med 2016; 95:407-415.

42. Zhang N, Zou Y, Jiang L, et al. Epstein Barr virus and neurologic diseases. Front Mol Biosci 2022; 10:1-34.

Index

OTHER BOOKS BY FOREST TENNANT

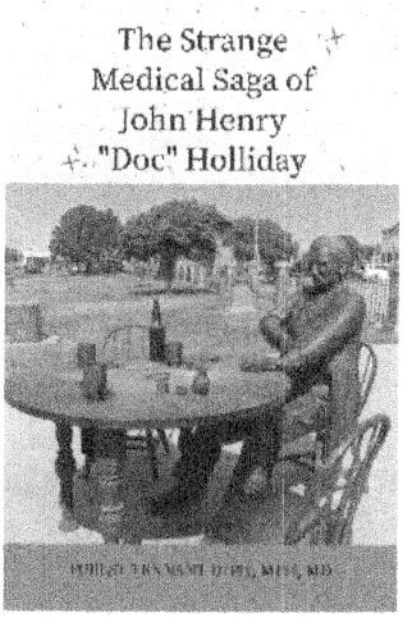

The Strange Medical Saga of "John Henry"
ISBN:9781955934275
LOC 2023913628

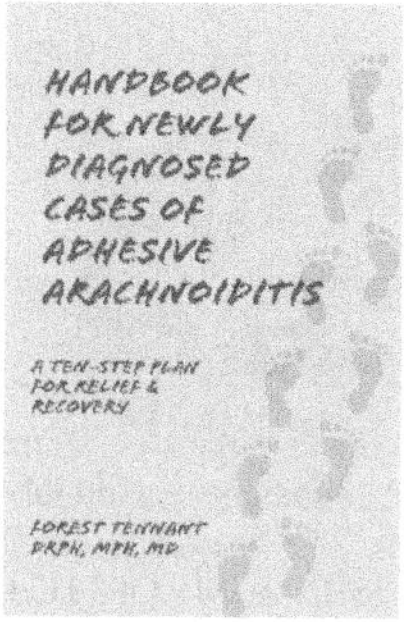

Handbook For Newly Diagnosed Cases of Adhesive Arachnoiditis
ISBN:9781955934244
LOC:2023908116

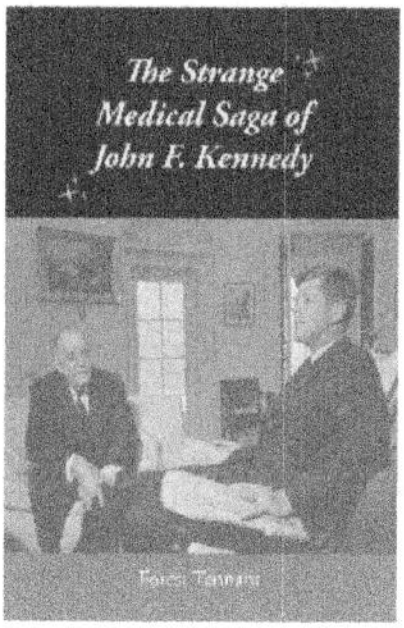

The Strange Medical Saga of JFK

ISBN:9781955934213
LOC:2023903440

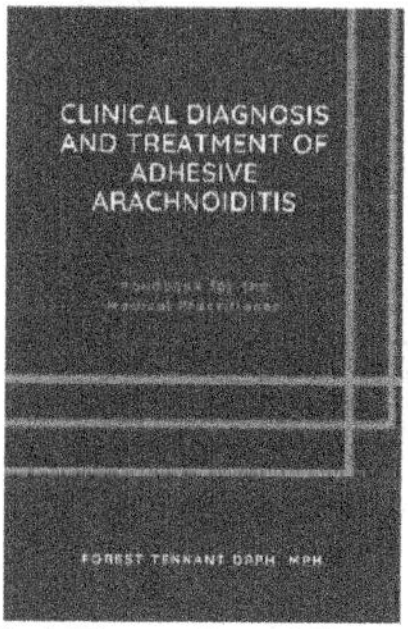

Clinical Diagnosis and Treatment of Adhesive Arachnoiditis
ISBN: 9781955934183
LOC: 2022907190

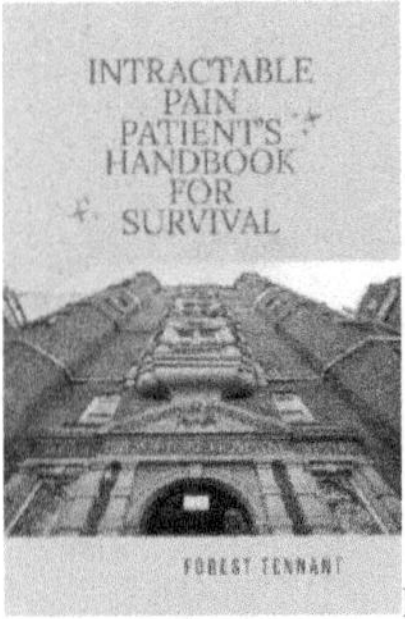

Intractable Pain Patients Handbook for Survival
ISBN: 9781955934121
LOC: 2021916464

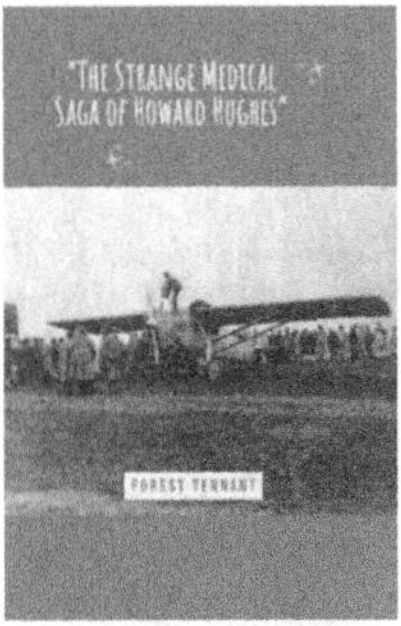

The Strange Medical Saga of Howard Hughes
ISBN: 9781955934091
LOC: 2021912855

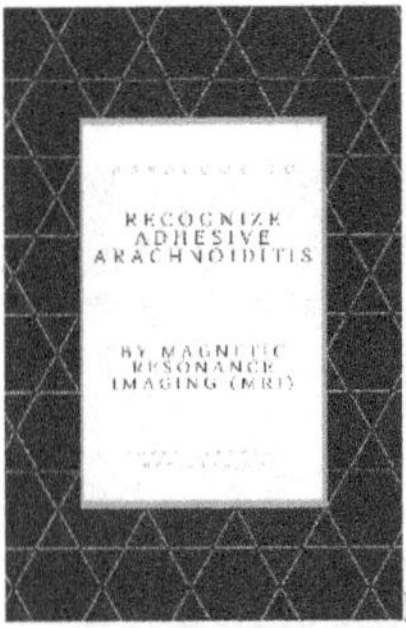

Handbook To Recognize Adhesive Arachnoiditis by Magnetic Resonance Imaging (MRI)
ISBN: 9781955934152
LOC: 2021925161

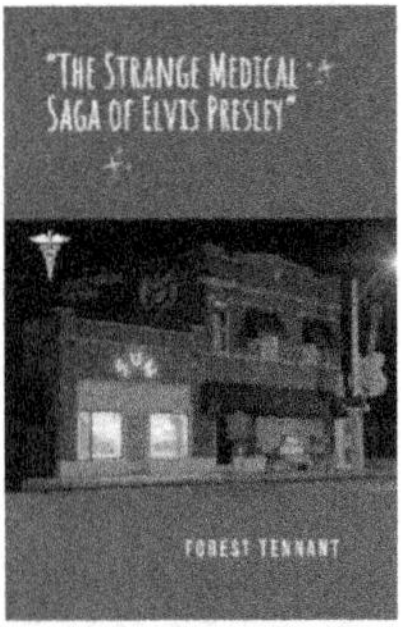

THE STRANGE MEDICAL SAGA OF ELVIS PRESLEY

ISBN: 9781955934008
LOC: 2021911718

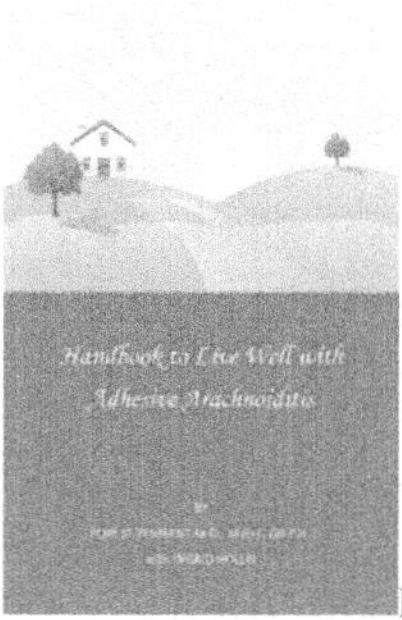

Handbook to Live Well with Adhesive Arachnoiditis

ISBN 978195934060
LOC: 2021912718

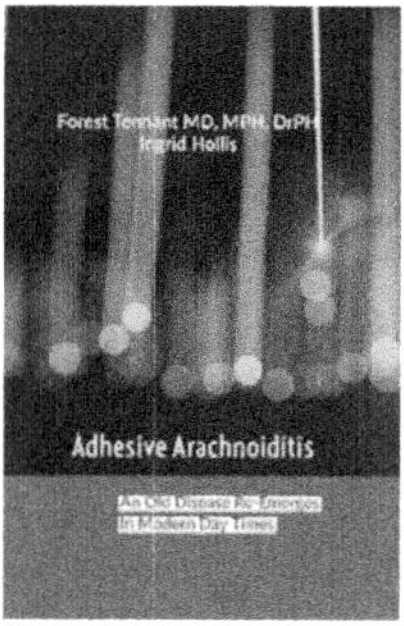

An Old Disease Re-Emerges in Modern Times

ISBN:9781955934039
LOC:2021912467

Made in the USA
Monee, IL
04 November 2026

67379305R00056